HOW TO GET FITTER AND STRONGER

A guide on how to burn calories, belly fat, add muscles, and keep FIT

DR BENJAMIN MICHEALS

Dr. Benjamin Micheals

TABLE OF CONTENTS

CHAPTER THREE

WAYS OF ACHIEVING FAT LOSS
EAT A LOT OF SOLUBLE FIBER
STAY AWAY FROM FOOD SOURCES THAT CONTAIN TRANS FATS
MODERATE YOUR LIQUOR CONSUMPTION
EAT A HIGH-PROTEIN DIET
LESSEN YOUR FEELINGS OF ANXIETY
TRY NOT TO EAT A LOT OF SWEET FOOD.
DO AEROBIC EXERCISES (CARDIO)
CUT BACK CARBS - PARTICULARLY REFINED CARBS
PERFORM RESISTANCE TRAINING (LIFT WEIGHTS)
LIMIT SUGAR-IMPROVED REFRESHMENTS
GET A LOT OF SOOTHING REST
TRACK YOUR FOOD INTAKE AND EXERCISE
EAT FATTY FISH CONSISTENTLY
LIMIT YOUR CONSUMPTION OF FRUIT JUICE
EAT PROBIOTIC FOOD VARIETIES OR TAKE A PROBIOTIC SUPPLEMENT
DRINK GREEN TEA
CHANGE YOUR WAY OF LIFE AND JOIN VARIOUS TECHNIQUES

CHAPTER FOUR

ASSEMBLING MUSCLE MASS
DEVELOPING MUSCLE
Increase Your Preparation Volume
Focus On the Eccentric Phase
Decrease Between-Set Rest Stretches
Eat More Protein
Focus On Calorie Surpluses
Nibble On Casein Before Bed
Get More Rest
Try supplementing With Creatine
Add HMB

CHAPTER FIVE

Dr. Benjamin Micheals

INTRODUCTION

Remaining fit is essentially as critical as the heart siphoning blood all through the body and the mind working to keep up with balance in our body. Being fit is the least we can do, inferable from the medical care circumstance and requirements winning presently. Various kinds of contamination and always rising infections debilitate the insusceptible framework. Youngsters are currently brought into the world with or determined to have sicknesses that prior used to strike people after their 40s. Subsequently, remaining fit and solid is currently a need to remain far away from such sicknesses. In this part, we'll be taking a gander at the fundamental necessities for staying in shape and solid. Diet, workout, and mental wellness are expected to accomplish positive outcomes toward being fit and solid, and solid.

CHAPTER 1

The Little Secrets

In our everyday activities, there are some habits I have termed the little secrets in our quest to lose weight, add muscles and keep fit.

Adjusted Diet

Food admission and dietary patterns assume a significant and prime part in the manner we carry on with our life and with what sort of way of life solid or undesirable. A fair eating regimen is of different constituents of food in precise and fitting amounts and quality as per the prerequisites of the person.

It is effectively edible and contains a fitting proportion between proteins, fats, and starches. The eating regimen might fluctuate from one individual to another as per the body's necessities.

A Dynamic Way of Life

This expects a significant part in staying aware of well-being. Schoolchildren ought to prefer strolling as opposed to being driven by a vehicle on the off chance that it is inside strolling distance. Steps can be utilized rather than lifts. Instead of adhering to television or versatile screens, one ought to choose outside games. As such, one could carry on with a more dynamic way of life.

Activities and Yoga

Research studies have demonstrated that pressure and strain lead to weight gain and ruin wellness levels. In this way, yoga and activities are important for keeping great control of weight and body wellness by consuming an overabundance of calories put away in your body and hence assume a huge part in keeping a solid weight when banded together with adjusted food.

Avoid Greasy Food Sources

Fats are a significant supporter of the quantity of calories. These additional numbers, which are more than the expected sum will quite often gather in the body. The more you try not to take them unreasonably, the better your possibilities of you staying fit. Likewise, abstain from gorging. The more food eaten, the more calories eaten past the body's prerequisites, consequently collection, in this way, expanding the body's possibilities of corpulence and way of life illnesses. Consuming inside the perfect amounts is better.

Try Not to Skip Supper Time

Skipping feasts is a severe no as against legends by people about eating fewer carbs for a fit body. When you skirt any dinner, you will go for gorging during the following feast time prompting weight gain, as this expands craving and results in more prominent food utilization sometime later.

Keep away from liquor, smoking, and medications
Continuously keep to you that these dependence specialists will quite often weight gain. Liquor is straightforwardly consumed from the stomach in the circulatory system and handily put away as fats. Stay away from it through and through to work with body wellness.

Dr. Benjamin Micheals

CHAPTER TWO

Legitimate propensities and schedules

We as a whole realize that there are numerous things we could do to work on our lives. In any case, it's a lot far from simple or easy.

That is the reason I'm proposing an alternate methodology. By placing things into the legitimate viewpoint, we can view our general well-being as a gathering of more modest propensities and schedules. Get these more modest propensities right and our general wellbeing makes certain to follow.

I've written this book to assist you with tracking down viable ways of getting more grounded and better. While there are no alternate routes, moving toward things the correct way is the main move toward begin characterizing your sound future. The schedules which were referenced in section one, are as per the following.

1. Work out
2. Diet
3. Mental wellness

At the point when dealt with together, these various regions can completely change you for a long-term benefit.

Work Out

It's notable that practice enormously upgrades one's personal satisfaction. In addition to the fact that the body delivers various strong synthetic substances that assuage pressure and support satisfaction while working out, however, it constructs muscle, bone thickness, and in general solidarity for sure!

Furthermore, exercise will help you look and feel your best, supporting your certainty and working on every one of the aspects of your life. We should take a gander at one or two workout schedules we can begin on immediately.

Cardio

Cardio offers phenomenal exercise for the entire body. It enhances muscle strength and the working of your heart and lungs.

It's ideal to do cardio a couple of days seven days for ideal outcomes. Certain individuals like doing it in the first part of the day while others lean toward night exercises that tire them out before bed. Analysis to find what works for yourself and stick with it.

However, I'd suggest stirring up your cardio preparation. From (HIIT) high-intensity interval training sessions to consistent state cardio.

Weight Lifting

Weight lifting is an extraordinary method for developing muscle fortitude and increment perseverance. The cycle works by building the muscles and bones through obstruction schedules. By rehashing these schedules again and again, the muscles tear and revamp, a characteristic interaction that leaves them better and more grounded over the long run.

Powerlifting is in many cases done several times each week (2x every week exercise). You can decide to do body-weight works out, powerlifting, or different other opposition exercises.

Adaptability Work Outs

This is one more extraordinary method for moulding the body. Adaptability exercises have detonated in prevalence throughout recent years because of the fair medical advantages they give.

For instance, yoga and jujitsu condition the body through the reiteration of specific body positions demonstrated to build flow, adaptability, and that's just the beginning.

Whether or not you might want to try different things with choices like yoga or judo, which are certain to consolidate extending and other delicate developments for well-being and generally body capability.

Diet

An appropriate eating routine is one more significant region to consider for the general strength of your body. You might have heard the expression - the type of food you eat will affect your general health. While this is to some degree a misnomer, the general message sounds valid.

The things you put in your body significantly affect your general working. And keeping in mind that many eating regimens have detonated onto the scene as of late, there are a couple of tips that everybody ought to follow for expanded well-being.

Cut Processed Sugar Intake

It's undeniably true that eating overabundance of processed sugar is terrible for your body. Think about cutting back desserts, and getting an apple or banana when the desire hit.

Increase Your Protein Intake

Your muscles require protein for development and support.

In this way, expanding your admission is a simple method for remaining solid. Eat loads of high-protein feasts and look at the steadily developing assortments of protein powders available.

Consume Leafy Foods

It's suggested that you eat something like 5 servings of leafy foods daily, however eating, significantly more, is a reliable method for remaining solid. Add verdant green vegetables and high-fiber choices for ideal nourishment.

Eat Standard Dinners

Food is fuel, and your body needs fuel to continue to function properly. Consider eating at customary spans to keep your body sustained and prepared to deal with the anxieties of life.

Drink A Lot of Water

Drinking sufficient water is a simple method for treating your body well. It's generally expected to hear that drinking 8 glasses a day is an incredible objective to go for the gold, exceeding all expectations by drinking up to 3 liters of water a day. It will truly assist with flushing out the poisons.

Placing the right things in your body is an unquestionable necessity for your drawn-out well-being and generally speaking strength.

Support your body and watch as different bits of your well-being plan get sorted out.

Since initially expounding on this point, I have been doing a ton of examination and perusing. I felt that I had passed up a part to do with the advantages of weight reduction.

There are countless non-visual advantages of shedding pounds, including:

- Diminished chance of diabetes
- Brought down circulatory strain
- Further developed cholesterol levels
- Diminished chance of coronary illness
- Diminished chance of specific tumours
- Further developed versatility
- Diminished joint torment
- Further developed glucose levels
- Diminished chance of stroke
- Diminished back torment
- Diminished hazard or improvement in side effects of osteoarthritis
- Diminished chance or improvement in side effects of rest apnea.

As may be obvious, there are countless advantages. Thus, while you're pondering getting in shape, look somewhat more profound than how your garments fit or how you thoroughly search in the mirror.

Mental Wellness

We've discussed keeping your body blissful and sound through practice and an appropriate eating routine. In any case, those are simply little bits of your general well-being and prosperity.
Your cerebrum requires its fuel as well, and proceeding to learn and work your psyche is significant for its life span and your general satisfaction. All things considered, a couple of everything things you can manage to remain intellectually sharp include:

Reading

Consider picking up a new book. Reading is a simple method for working your brain and engaging yourself simultaneously.

Journaling

Current life is distressing, and journaling can be an incredible delivery. Consider writing your contemplations down to assist you with figuring out them or use WordPress (it's a free publishing content to a blog programming stage).

Taking a Class

Regardless of whether you've finished school, there are various on the web and one-time classes you can take to remain sharp.

Testing Yourself

Challenge yourself to attempt new things. Our minds like to remain in their usual ranges of familiarity, yet that is not the way in which we develop. Investigate new spots and think about additional opportunities, and watch as your brain grows.

These are only a couple of tips to consider, however, there are a lot more out there! Utilize your creative mind to find things that rouse you to learn and develop. It's hard, however, it's worth the effort.

Keep at It

We've viewed the three best ways of remaining fit, sound, areas of strength and for the years to come. Simply recall that it requires investment and commitment to see the progressions you need.

Consider the purposes for why you need to treat yourself well, and afterward stay with it! You should be fit, sound, serious areas of strength and, you can begin to see positive outcomes in a matter of moments.

CHAPTER THREE

Ways of Achieving Fat Loss

An excessive amount of belly fat can increase your chances of some chronic conditions. Drinking less liquor, eating more protein, and lifting loads are only a couple of steps you can take to lose belly fat.

Having an overabundance of belly fat can adversely influence well-being and may add to a few ongoing circumstances.

One explicit kind of belly fat that is; visceral fat, is a significant risk factor for type 2 diabetes, coronary illness, and different circumstances. Numerous health organizations use body mass index (BMI) to group weight and predict the risk of metabolic illness.

Nonetheless, BMI is just determined utilizing height and weight and doesn't consider body composition or visceral fat.

However, losing fat from this area can be troublesome, there are a few things you can do to decrease the overabundance of stomach fat.

The following are 17 viable tips to lose belly fat.

Eat a Lot of Soluble Fiber

Soluble fiber ingests water and forms a gel that slows down food as it goes through your stomach.

This fiber will advance weight reduction by assisting you with feeling full, so you normally eat less.

Hence, soluble fiber assist with diminishing tummy fat.

Phenomenal sources of soluble fiber include:

- Fruits
- Legumes
- Vegetables
- Oats

- Grain

Generally, soluble fiber might assist you with getting in shape by expanding completion and lessening calorie assimilation. Try to include a lot of high-fiber food varieties for your eating routine.

Stay Away from Food Sources That Contain Trans Fats

Trans fats are made by adding hydrogen into unsaturated fats, for example, soybean oil.

Already, they were tracked down in certain margarine and spreads and furthermore frequently added to packaged food varieties, however, most food makers have quit utilizing them.

These fats have been connected to the aggravation of coronary illness, and insulin obstruction.

To assist with lessening stomach fat, read the ingredient label carefully and avoid items that contain trans fats.

Moderate Your Liquor Consumption

Liquor can have medical advantages in limited quantities, however, it tends to be destructive in the event that you drink excessively, as expressed in past chapters.

An excess of liquor can add to belly fat.

Reducing liquor intake might assist with lessening your belly fat. You don't have to surrender it totally, yet restricting the sum you drink in a solitary day can help.

As indicated by the latest Dietary Rules for Americans, it's prescribed to restrict liquor admission to two drinks or less each day for men and one drink or less each day for ladies.

Excessive liquor intake has been related to increased belly fat. In the event that you are attempting to get thinner, think about savouring liquor control or going without totally.

Eat a High-Protein Diet

Protein is a critical supplement for weight control.

High protein consumption increases the release of the fullness hormone peptide YY, which diminishes hunger and promotes fullness.

Protein likewise raises your metabolic rate and assists you with retaining muscle mass during weight reduction.

People who eat more protein will regularly have less stomach fat than individuals who eat a lower protein diet. Make sure to incorporate a decent protein source at each dinner, for example,

- Meat
- Fish
- Eggs
- Dairy
- Whey protein
- Beans

Lessen Your Feelings of Anxiety

Stress can make you gain tummy fat by setting off the adrenal organs to deliver cortisol, otherwise called the pressure chemical.

High cortisol levels increase hunger and drive stomach fat capacity.

Likewise, ladies who as of now have a large waist will generally produce more cortisol in response to stress. Increased cortisol levels further add to fat addition.

To assist with decreasing belly fat, participate in exercises that reduce pressure. Rehearsing yoga or meditation can be effective.

Try Not to Eat a Lot of Sweet Food.

Sugar might contain fructose, which is connected to a few ongoing sicknesses when consumed in high quantities.

These include coronary illness, type 2 diabetes, and fatty liver infections.

It's essential to understand that refined sugar can increase fat. Indeed, even regular sugars, like genuine honey, ought to be utilized in moderation.

Excess sugar intake is a significant reason for weight gain in many individuals. Limit your intake of candy and food varieties high in added sugar.

Do Aerobic Exercises (Cardio)

Aerobic exercise (cardio) is a viable method for improving your well-being and burn calories.

It very well may be a successful type of activity for diminishing belly fat. Nonetheless, results are mixed with regard to whether moderate or high-intensity exercise is more valuable.

Anyway, the frequency and length of your activity program can likewise be vital.

High-impact exercise is a viable weight reduction strategy.

Cut Back Carbs - Particularly Refined Carbs

Reducing your carb intake can be extremely advantageous for losing fat, including belly fat.

As a matter of fact, low-carb diets might cause belly fat loss in individuals with overweight, those in danger of type 2 diabetes, and individuals with polycystic ovary condition (PCOS).

You don't need to follow a severe low-carb diet. Refined carbs with unprocessed starchy carbs may work on metabolic well-being and lessen belly fat.

A high intake of refined carbs is related to excessive belly fat. Consider decreasing your carb intake or replacing refined carbs in your eating regimen with sound carb sources, like whole grains, legumes, or vegetables.

Perform Resistance Training (Lift Weights)

Resistance training, otherwise called weightlifting or strength training, is significant for preserving and acquiring mass.

For individuals with prediabetes, type 2 diabetes, and fatty liver diseases, resistance training may likewise be valuable for belly fat misfortune.

As a matter of fact, teens with overweight showed a blend of strength, and aerobic exercise prompted the best reduction in visceral fat.

In the event that you choose to begin lifting loads, it's really smart to converse with a specialist first and get advice from a guaranteed fitness coach.

Strength training can be a significant weight reduction system and may assist with decreasing belly fat. It's considerably more effective mixed with aerobic exercise.

Limit Sugar-Improved Refreshments

Sugar-improved refreshments are high in added sugars like fructose, which can add to stomach fat.

Individuals with type 2 diabetes found that consuming something like one serving of sugar-improved drinks each week was related to increased belly fat compared to consuming less than one serving each week.

Furthermore, in light of the fact that your brain doesn't deal with liquid calories the same way it does solid ones, you're probably going to wind up consuming an excessive number of calories later on and taking care of them as fat.

To lose belly fat, it's ideal to restrict your intake of sugar-improved refreshments, for example,

- Soda
- Punch
- Sweet tea
- Alcohol mixers containing sugar

Get a Lot of Soothing Rest

Rest is significant for some parts of your well-being, including weight. Not getting sufficient rest is connected to a higher risk of obesity and increased belly fat.

The condition known as sleep apnea, where breathing stops irregularly during the night, has additionally been connected to an abundance of visceral fat.

As well as resting for something like 7 hours in the evening, ensure you're getting adequate quality rest.

In the event that you suspect you have sleep apnea or another rest problem, think about addressing a specialist regarding treatment choices.

Track Your Food Intake and Exercise

Numerous things can assist you with getting fitter and losing belly fat, yet consuming fewer calories than your body needs for weight upkeep is vital.

Keeping a food journal or utilizing a web-based food tracker or application can assist with checking your calorie consumption. This procedure has been demonstrated to be helpful for weight reduction.

Moreover, food tracking tools assist you with seeing your intake of protein, carbs, fiber, and micronutrients. Many additionally permit you to record your activity and actual work.

You can find a few free applications or sites to track nutrient and calorie consumption.

Eat Fatty Fish Consistently

Fatty fish can be a nutritious expansion to a reasonable eating routine.

They're wealthy in top-notch protein and omega-3 fats which offer assurance against persistent illness.

Some proof recommends that these omega-3 fats may likewise assist with reducing visceral fat.

Get at least 2 servings of fatty fish each week. Good choices include:

- Salmon
- Herring
- Sardines
- Mackerel
- anchovies

For veggie lovers, vegans, and individuals who don't consistently consume fish, plant-based omega-3 enhancements got from sources like algae are also available.

Limit Your Consumption of Fruit Juice

In spite of the fact that organic product juice gives nutrients and minerals, it's generally expected similarly as high in sugar as soda and other improved refreshments.

For instance, an 8-ounce (248-milliliter) serving of unsweetened squeezed apple contains 24 g of sugar, over half of which is fructose.

Drinking high measures of organic product juice could add to weight gain because of the unnecessary measure of calories that it gives instead of the fructose that it contains.

All things considered, to assist with decreasing excessive belly fat, moderate your intake of sugary drinks by appreciating different drinks with lower sugar content, like water, unsweetened chilled tea, or shimmering water with a wedge of lemon or lime.

Eat Probiotic Food Varieties or Take a Probiotic Supplement

Probiotics are microorganisms tracked down in certain food varieties and enhancements. They have medical advantages, including further developing gut well-being and improving the immune system.

Be that as it may, while probiotics might be valuable for weight reduction, more exploration is required. As certain probiotics aren't controlled by the Food and Medication Organization, it's essential to converse with a specialist prior to adding probiotics or different enhancements to your daily schedule.

Taking probiotic improvements could help with propelling a sound stomach-related system. There is likewise advantageous stomach microbiota that might assist with advancing weight reduction.

Drink Green Tea

Green tea is an outstandingly sound drink.

It contains caffeine and the antioxidant epigallocatechin gallate (EGCG), which seems to support digestion.

EGCG is a catechin, which will assist you with losing belly fat. The effect may be supported when green tea use is joined together with work out.

Green tea increases weight reduction, particularly when consumed in dosages of under 500 milligrams each day for a long time.

Change Your Way of Life and Join Various Techniques

Doing one of the things on this rundown might not hugely affect its own.

For best outcomes, consolidating various techniques might be more powerful.

Curiously, a considerable lot of these techniques are by and largely connected with adjusted eating and an in general solid way of life.

In this manner, changing your way of life for the long haul is the way to lose your belly fat and keep it off.

At the point when you have solid propensities, remain dynamic, and lessen your intake of ultra-handled food. Fat loss will in general follow as a characteristic secondary effect.

The primary concern

There are no enchanted answers for losing belly fat.

Weight reduction generally requires some work, responsibility, and determination.

Embracing some of the systems as a whole and way of life objectives examined in this article will assist you with losing paunch fat and working on general well-being.

Dr. Benjamin Micheals

CHAPTER FOUR

Assembling Muscle Mass

Patience is misinterpreted, particularly in the weight room. At the point when there's ordinarily a particular wanted result for competitors: sorting out some way to construct muscle.

Certainly, change takes time. In any case, in the event that you're attempting to track down the quickest method for developing muscle and aren't seeing clear size increments from one month to another, it's a sign your methodology is off.

Besides, regardless of whether you are seeing improvement, there's no great explanation you can't endeavour to see more solid additions.

How would you fire up your outcomes? The following are nine hints that will show you how to assemble muscle.

Developing Muscle

Increase Your Preparation Volume

Your number of reps copied by your number of sets is a fundamental determiner of hypertrophy (muscle volume advancement). What's more, to increase volume, you may really have to go lower in weight than you could figure.

Contrasted with preparing for strength, power will drop during the hypertrophy period of a program, with power sitting somewhere in the range of 50 and 75 percent of the individual's 1RM (one rep-max), the most extreme weight the person can lift for one rep.

To get the volume your muscles need, I recommend playing out all of your lifts for three to six plans of 10 to 20 reps.

Focus on the Eccentric Phase

While lifting any weight, you will have a concentric (agonist muscle contracting) and flighty (bad guy muscle extending stage).

For example, as you lower into a squat, you're playing out an unpredictable activity. Exactly when you return to standing, that is concentric. Unpredictable work is far superior at setting off hypertrophy.

To expand how much unpredictable exertion is in your exercise, you can complete two things: either delayed down the flighty period of each exercise you perform or coordinate erratic just varieties into your everyday exercise.

Take the squat, for instance. To make it eccentric-only, you would lower to the floor, and end the exercise there. Note: Assuming you're attempting eccentric-only exercises, you'll have to considerably increase the weight that you use. Physiologically, muscles are far more grounded moving eccentrically than they are concentric.

Decrease Between-Set Rest Stretches

Assuming that you contact your telephone between practice sets, it should be to set its clock to 30 to 90 seconds.

While lifting for hypertrophy, rest times of 30 to 90 seconds support a fast delivery of muscle-building chemicals (counting testosterone and human development chemical) while likewise ensuring that you, as a matter of fact, genuinely fatigue your muscles.

Regardless of rep and set plot, exhausting your muscles is essential for hypertrophy.

Make sure to feel the burn.

Eat More Protein

Strength training separates your muscles, and protein constructs them back up. The more troublesome your lifting exercises are, the more significant muscle-building food sources become while gauging protein intake to cement recuperation.

For a 175-pound individual, that works out, 20 to 24 grams of protein at each meal.

You'll get that in around three to four eggs, a glass of Greek yogurt, or one scoop of protein powder.

Focus on Calorie Surpluses

This can be a hard one to become acclimated to, particularly for people who are accustomed to including calories with expectations of destroying fat. In any case, with regards to how to acquire bulk quickly (that implies weight acquired, not lost), you want to consume a bigger number of calories than you consume every day.

That is on the grounds that, when your body detects that it's in a calorie deficiency — importance you're consuming fewer calories than you're burning every day — it downshifts your body's propensity to fabricate new muscle. All things considered, assuming your body thinks food is hard to come by, getting swollen won't be its primary need.

Meaning to eat approximately 250 to 500 additional calories each day. To ensure that any weight acquired is from muscle. The bulk of those calories should come from protein

Nibble on Casein Before Bed

Long well-known among bodybuilders, casein proteins ingest gradually into the circulatory system, meaning it keeps your muscles fed with amino acids for longer compared with different sorts of protein, like whey and plant proteins. Consuming casein protein preceding bed time boosted young men's degrees of circulating amino acids for 7.5 hours. They fabricated muscle the entire night while they rested.

To get some pre-bed time casein, attempt curds(cheese), Greek yogurt, and milk.

For smoothie lovers, casein-based protein powder has exactly the intended effect.

Get More Rest

Muscle recuperation requires more than the right sustenance. It requires investment — around eight hours out of every evening — committed to recuperation. In light of everything, when you rest, your body releases an anabolic compound, which creates muscle and holds levels of the tension synthetic cortisol inside legitimate cutoff points.

Resting for five hours, rather than eight hours each night for only one week cuts muscle-building testosterone levels by an astounding 10 to 15%.

Hence, grown-ups age 18 to 64 should rest eight to nine hours out of every evening.

Try Supplementing with Creatine

Creatine doesn't directly develop muscle. However, they boost your performances at high level work out lifting exercises, the natural compound increases muscle development.

At a given weight, upgrading with creatine can help you with lifting 14% a greater number of reps than you can. For the best outcomes, select creatine monohydrate, the most completely explored type of enhancement.

Add HMB

A characteristic compound produced in the human body, beta-hydroxy-beta-methylbutyrate forestalls muscle-protein breakdown, empowers muscle development, and speeds exercise recuperation.

Tragically, it's difficult to fundamentally increase levels through food alone. That is where supplementation comes in.

Additionally, in case you propel yourself excessively hard, HMB forestalls the impacts of overtraining including muscle loss.

To help your endeavors to develop muscle, you can take HMB supplements solo or choose protein and creatine powders that come with HMB prepared right in.

CHAPTER FIVE

Maintaining a Healthy Body Composition

Envision you have arrived at your weight reduction objectives
Also, presently you are hoping to keep up with your body weight and the muscles you have acquired. What do you do?

That is the very thing that body composition exercises are there for. It might seem confounded; however, a portion of these body creation practices are essentially straightforward, when joined with a reasonable and sound eating regimen, you will not only maintain but strengthen your body as well.

Above all, how about we comprehend what body composition is? Body composition is what your body is comprised of, be it muscle, bones, or fat. A fair body composition comprises a diminished level of body fats and a higher level of non-fat mass, which consolidates muscle, bones, and organs.

Why stress over body structure and not simply weight? I'm certain if you acquired muscle, and the number on the scale increases, you probably won't be aware assuming it's fat or muscle. That is the reason taking a gander at body structure is significant and supportive.

What are good body fat percentage levels?

For men, the ideal body fat percentage is between 18-24%, and for ladies, it is 25-31%. These numbers, in any case, are probably going to change contingent on the individual's age and well-being.

Suggested Body Composition Exercises.

Here are a bunch of exercises that focus on your whole body. A compelling method for executing a total body creation practice is by arranging targeted - push-ups, burpees, rushes, and squat leaps and boards as a feature of an intense cardio exercise (HIIT) program.

Body composition is a preferable measure overweight. The objective isn't to get into a lifting weights exercise and gym routine however a designated preparation to burn calories and trigger muscle development and keep up with consistency by keeping your pulse high by keeping away from long breaks between

Workouts

Perfect combinations for exercises.

Combine your most loved cardio exercises with strength training and alternate between them in a solitary exercise. For instance, you could do a mix of running, cycling, and climbing a slope for 5 minutes each, then push-ups and stomach crunches for 5 minutes each. Repeat this example 3-6 times for complete high-intensity exercise.

Alternating your exercises on various days additionally assists you to maximize your training while permitting your body an adequate chance to recuperate. For instance, on Mondays, Wednesdays, and Fridays you could zero in on strength training while at the same time utilizing Tuesdays and Thursdays to zero in on cardio, extending, and recuperation.

It's vital to get both cardio and strength preparing exercises into your daily schedule, as both convey unique, yet similarly significant, results.

The following are five extraordinary exercises you can do at home to hold your body structure within proper limits. Prior to endeavouring any of these activities, on the off chance that you are having any unexpected problems it is encouraged to talk with your coach and specialist first.

Burpee

Performing Burpees is an amazing method for preparing both cardio perseverance and strength. Many consider Burpees as the best all-out body practice as they utilize each muscle in the body, including the heart. You will find that these work your leg muscles, core, and even shoulders. A squat, a push-up, and a leap are completely remembered for a Burpee. They're additionally not suggested for those with back issues.

Push-Ups

This exercise is suggested by specialists as a superior option in contrast to utilizing a chest press machine. It is on the grounds that it assists you with developing your muscles and actuates your entire core simultaneously. They are especially valuable in strong development, despite the fact that they are not the most straightforward. The chest, legs, shoulder, arms, and core muscles will be generally worked out in this total body workout.

Squats

Squats are a brilliant activity for holding your body creation within proper limits. They're particularly great for working out the muscles in your lower body. Assuming that you wear a weighted vest, it can truly help your exercise by adding that additional load to fortify your legs.

Planks

planks are another astounding body arrangement exercise that you can add to your exercise routine daily schedule. The practice is especially valuable in further developing stance by fortifying various muscles like the core, shoulders, hamstrings, and glutes.

Ab Targeting

For some, most of their fat is held around the stomach, yet, doing more abdominal muscle moves isn't the best method for diminishing the fat there. Having said that, it's as yet essential and prescribed to integrate some abdominal muscle moves into your exercises to reinforce the core and fabricate those muscles. Moreover, you can include numerous moves finished one after the other, for example, hanging leg raises, side planks, stomach muscle crunches, and bike crunches. Also, don't disregard the back muscles, so moves like dorsal raises will assist with that.

Top Tips

The key is to get going gradually so you don't wear out. Indeed, even a little 15-minute exercise will assist you with getting to the next level. Then, at that point, as you progress you can build the force and length of your exercises.
The best way to accomplish results is consistency. Assuming you train regularly, build up to 4 sessions per week, and proceed with that daily practice for 5 months and you will see excellent results.

This might sound overwhelming consolidating cardio HIIT with strength and resistance training, yet everything will stream flawlessly once you see the distinction in each activity. A devoted daily schedule, a consistent approach, and a balanced diet are what it takes.

Dr. Benjamin Micheals

53

CONCLUSION

In the quest to lose weight, diet is as important as the exercises that are carried out. Exercising without the required or proper dieting will not yield favourable results. For example, excess calories in the body are stored as fat. Hence, calories must be taken in the appropriate amounts as you embark on exercises to reduce body weight and add muscle mass, depending on what you require.

Being healthy and fit also saves you from some diseases associated with obesity, so we should endeavour to live a fit and healthy lifestyle.

www.ingramcontent.com/pod-product-compliance
Lightning Source LLC
Chambersburg PA
CBHW051356250726
48656CB00006B/2121